NO EXCUSES!

Day 1/ Date_____
Good morning.
Read today's motivation.

Begin by taking as many measurements and stats as possible. We have been so programmed, to watch the scale, that we can get discouraged if the number does not move fast enough or in the right direction. When we have lots of numbers, we can see that we are still progressing even if the weight number does not move.

We have talked about choosing a nutrition plan that suits you. That means looking for a plan or designing a plan that takes into account your habits and your food likes. Anything else is just a diet.

It has been proven that a reduction in calories, under what your body uses during the day, will result in weight loss. That calorie restriction can come from any part of your nutrition… fats, carbohydrates, or protein. Be careful that you do not restrict a food group so severely, that it backfires in a binge down the road. Moderate, long term weight loss and fitness will result in a life time of enjoyment, versus a fad diet that results in you gaining even more weight when you can't maintain the lifestyle.

Fill out the SMART GOAL WORKSHEET. Be as detail specific as you can about where you want to be. Believe in yourself.

DAY # 1/ Date: _____

SMART GOAL SETTING

SPECIFIC: What is your goal? Be specific. Answer WHO?
WHAT? WHEN? WHERE? HOW?

_____

_____

_____

List 3 specific steps to take to reach your goal.

1.)_____

2.)_____

3.)_____

MEASUREABLE:

How you will track your goal?

_____

How you will measure your progress?

_____

What does your progress look like?

_____

ATTAINABLE:

What can you do to make this goal achievable?

_____

What resources do you need?

_____

What support system do you need?

_____

What items do you need to make this work?

_____

How can you make this work?

_____

RELEVANT:

How will your life change when you reach your goal?

_____

What will happen if you do not reach this goal?

_____

TIMELY: What is your time line and breakdown of the different steps involved in reaching your goal?

_____

_____

_____

_____

PUT YOUR GOALS IN YOUR TRAINING LOGBOOK

**Comments and
Notes:** _____

_____

_____

_____

Day 2/ Date_____
Good Morning,
Read your motivation for today.

You can see, that even with some goals it's going to be important to fine tune your plan. It's time to take action.

Fill out the PLAN OF ACTION, to help you narrow down what your habits are now, and how you can change the areas that are weak into something that works.

The idea is to FAIL FAST.
Nobody is perfect. That's why we are logging our nutrition. You bought the book, now take the time to follow through. No excuses. That's just a way to allow your self to slide back into old habits. People who log tend to have better results then those who don't. It makes you accountable for your actions. It allows you to see patterns that are destructive. It pinpoints areas that are not working so that you fail fast and quickly re-plan your strategy for success.

You are unlike anyone else on earth. You need to be able to see what works for you as an individual.

NOW TAKE ACTION:
Based on your own plan, prepare your foods for the day. Plan meals for the coming week and gather your supplies. NO EXCUSES. You have the ability to do this. As you do your exercise, record it in your logbook. When you have a good day of nutrition, mark a line on the FOOD/EXERCISE page. Put another line when you eat healthy.

Use the WEEKLY MEAL PLAN to think ahead about what

events are coming up in your life, and what you intend to eat. And plan what your go to meal replacement will be if you can't get to your meal.

Day #2/ Date:_____

<u>PLAN OF ACTION</u>

What is your daily eating schedule? Look for patterns and problem areas. What times do you eat at and what type of food do you reach for?

_____
_____
_____
_____
_____
_____
_____
_____
_____
_____
_____
_____
_____
_____
_____
_____
_____

What is your nutritional plan now? Times of eating and plan of action? How will you substitute for the foods that are your triggers? What can you put in place of the habitual snacking times?

_____
_____
_____
_____
_____

How can you make sure you have the foods you need prepared for when you need them? When can you prepare foods? How often does this need to happen? What about when you are traveling or it's the weekend?

_____

_____
_____
_____
_____
_____
_____

How often will you workout? What will you do for exercise? How can you make sure you get to all workouts? What days and times will you make available to get exercise?

_____
_____
_____
_____
_____
_____
_____

PUT YOUR BASIC PLAN INTO YOUR LOG BOOK NOTES. PUT REMINDERS OF TIMES ON YOUR SCHEDULE OR CALENDAR. LEAVE STICKY NOTES TO TRIGGER YOURSELF TO FOLLOW THROUGH. **NO EXCUSES!**

Day 3/ Date_____
Good Morning,
Read your motivation for the day,

We often say things to ourselves that we would never say to someone else. We seem to be our own worst critics. And guess what? We believe ourselves.

Bottom line…you are unique, fearfully, and wonderfully created. It's time to stop filling our own heads with nonsense.

Fill out OUR INNER DIALOGUE. Pay attention to what we think about ourselves and how we talk about ourselves through out the day. Try to replace these negatives with a positive spin.

Remember your motto….NO EXCUSES.

***Talk to yourself positively
***Chart your foods…and be honest
***Chart your exercise.
***Look at your meals and try to find healthy replacements for those areas of your day that seem to have unhealthy choices. Fail fast and fix the problem.

OUR INNER DIALOGUE

List three negative things you tell yourself:
1)_____
2)_____
3)_____

List three things you can possitively say to
yourself , instead of the negative.
1)_____
2)_____
3)_____

List three positive things that you like about
yourself.
1)_____
2)_____
3)_____

Day 4/ Date_____
Good Morning,
Read your motivation for the day,

Don't be afraid to take your picture. Others see you every day. This is just another tool to assess where you are coming from, and determine where you are going. You wouldn't travel across country without a map, so don't expect to get to where you want to be without a clear vision. This doesn't need to be in a bathing suit. Just wear a normal pair of your clothes that plainly shows your body. (Tank top and jeans, etc)

Paste front/side/and back before pictures in your workbook. (That's what we are going to be working on) Paste an additional front picture into the back of your log book.

Find a picture of someone who has the same build as you (possibly even a picture from an earlier time when you were fit), then put your head on the new picture. This is the vision you have to look at for 'Where You Are Going'.

Don't worry. You don't ever plan on being this unfit again. Believe in yourself. You are strong.

Day #4/ Date:_____ **PICTURES**

Paste before pictues here. Add one to your logbook. Attach your head
to a picture of the body you want to give you motivation for where you are going.

Front Before

Back Before

Side Before

Picture of where
you are going

Day 5/ Date_____

Good Morning,

Read your motivation for the day,

People who build vision boards or find ways to envision their results, are more successful at achieving their goals than those who don't.

Write down what you want your life to look like. Draw a picture of that costume you want to wear for Halloween, paste pictures of that vacation you want to go on. The more real your future life is, the quicker it will come to you.

The things we do in this book are important because they make you think and keep you engaged in your journey. NO EXCUSES. Do the exercises and stay involved.

We have lived our lives for years doing the same things out of habit. It is important for us to work hard to recreate new habits. Stick with the program and follow through. You are worth it.

My Vision

Write down, draw, or paste pictures of how
you envision your life to be.

Day 6/ Date_____
Good Morning,
Read your motivation for the day,

You often hear people wonder why someone can't lose weight by just changing or reducing their eating. Because most weight issues are not as much about hunger, as being emotionally connected to food.

Fill out EMOTIONAL EATING.

Some people eat for any emotional reason, and others eat for particular reasons. It's important to know how you react to different emotions.

Our environments are in a constant state of change. There will always be death and birth, weddings and funerals, happy times and sad times. When we are aware of how we are affected, we can choose the way we react.

Emotional eating

What is your pattern when you first become emotional?

_____

_____

_____

Which type of emotions trigger negative behavior?

Name 3 situations that could crop up and how you could handle them differently than by over eating.

_____

_____

_____

_____

_____

_____

Day 7
Good Morning,
Read your motivation for the day,

Weekends are harder for most people to stay committed. That means it's even more important to plan ahead possible stumbling blocks.

Look at your food log. Make a list of times that you were thrown off course and what caused it.
Figure out what events are coming for the weekend.
Plan a course of action to cover any event (going out, staying in, etc.)

It's fine to have a cheat meal if that's part of your plan. It's ok to have foods you love if you prepare it healthy ahead of time in the right amounts. But it's not ok to decide to wing it. Where has that gotten you before?

You got out of shape by not thinking. It takes hard work and thinking to retrain yourself to get back in shape. Stick with it. You are worth it.

Day#7/Date:_____

WEEKEND PLAN

Look at your log book and note what time/event/triggers messed up your nutritional plan. Then decide on a corrective plan of action to help you through the weekend without derailing.

Time	Event	Trigger

SATURDAY EVENTS AND FOOD PLAN:

_____

_____

_____

_____

SUNDAY EVENTS AND FOOD PLAN:

_____

_____

_____

_____

DAY 8/Date:_____
Good morning.
Read your motivation for the day.
<u>Nutrition</u>
Let's talk nutrition. Fad diets typically don't work because they limit certain foods and people are unable to sustain that type of eating as a forever lifestyle.

It doesn't matter which food group you limit (Carbohydrates/Protein/Fats), if you take in less calories than you use, you will lose weight. However, if you eliminate a group entirely, you can also limit nutrients that your body may need.

Bottom line…if you eat what your creator provides us, in balanced portions, you tend to stay healthier. When your body eats too much processed foods (crackers, cookies, donuts, candy, etc), your body says, "What the heck is this?" It has no nutritional value.

Finding a plan that involves all the food groups, in moderation, can provide good health as well as weight loss.

<u>Macronutrients should fall in the following ranges:</u>
***Protein…….……10-35% of total calories
***Fat……….……… 20-35% of total calories
***Carbohydrate…..45-65%of total calories

FILL OUT YOUR WEEKLY MENU PLAN. MAKE ADJUSTMENTS TO BALANCE OUT YOUR MEALS. EATING A PROTEIN/A CARB/AND SOME VEGGIES AT EACH MEAL CAN MEET THESE REQUIREMENTS.

MODIFICATIONS TO YOUR MEALS

List some of your favorite foods that you would be sad to live without. Then figure out how you can make a healthier version and add it into your weekly plan. (Caution; A good plan can sometimes mean making just enough to have a serving, then saving a serving for a different meal and finishing off with vegetables. That way you don't overeat by creating too much).

FAVORITE MEALS   MADE HEALTHIER

_____

_____

_____

_____

_____

_____

_____

_____

_____

_____

_____

_____

Day 9/ Date_____
Good morning.
Read your motivation for the day.

Did you fill out your WEEKLY NOTES in your log?
The purpose of using your weekly notes is to find out where
you have gaps and tweak your action plan to cover any gaps.
For instance; you knew you were going to dinner and thought
you'd just have a salad. When you got there, all of the salads
looked so good that you just went with the Taco Salad with
sour crème, olives, and deep fried shell.

You could call this your cheat meal. You could realize that the
extra unplanned calories are part of that 20% nutrition that
we don't do well and forgive yourself. You could also realize
that regardless of how good or bad you ate, the meal is now
history and it's time to move on.

However, you might also remember that unplanned eating is
how you got into this mess. A better plan of future action
would be to Google the restaurant menu, or stop by before you
went out, and know *exactly* what you want to order and where
it fits in your nutrition plan for the day. Then look ahead in
your action plan and menus to tweak anything that needs
better planning.

Fill out the Energy Output Form each day this week.
Note when you have energy changes. Then put the same meal
in at the same time, on a different day, but change the amount
of protein or carbs to see if your energy output feel better.

And FINALLY: You have spent a life of creating habits. To
change those habits, there may be a need to create and
artificial prodding. Set your alarm to remind you to eat on
time. Set additional alarms and leave notes to remind you to

chart and recheck any actions you need to do on your menu plan each day.

You got into this situation by not thinking. You have to have a plan to create change.

Energy output: Chart either high energy or low		
Time	Meal	Results
Mon		
Tues		
Wed		
Thurs		
Fri		
Sat		
Notes:		

Energy output: Chart either high energy or low

Time	Meal	Results
Mon		
Tues		
Wed		
Thurs		
Fri		
Sat		
Notes:		

Energy output: Chart either high energy or low

Time	Meal	Results
Mon		
Tues		
Wed		
Thurs		
Fri		
Sat		
Notes:		

Energy output: Chart either high energy or low

Time	Meal	Results
Mon		
Tues		
Wed		
Thurs		
Fri		
Sat		
Notes:		

Day 10/ Date_____
Good morning.
Read your motivation.

When looking at food choices…all choices are not equal. You might have a choice of a donut or scrambled eggs with toast. While both choices may have the same calories, the scrambled eggs with toast will provide longer term satisfaction, energy, and nutritional quality than the donut.

When we talk about eating well 80% of the time and not worrying about things the other 20% of the time, we still have too have a plan in place.

For instance: You pay your rent, utilities, car payment, and etcetera first, then you can use left over money to put on vacation and fun. The same goes for your nutrition. You plan healthy meals and snacks to meet your energy, health, and physical needs. Then you PLAN when you can allow the occasional fun food to come along. You have a cheat meal each week. That's part of your action plan and you can indulge with no guilt, knowing the rest of the week you ate healthy and on schedule. Or you plan a piece of birthday cake or a Thanksgiving meal into your week, knowing those calories are coning up, and adjusting accordingly. It's the not thinking and planning that gets us into a habit of wreaking our program continually.

Fast food and restaurants are a normal lifestyle for many working people on the go. Good choices can be made if you plan in advance to where you are going.

TIPS for eating out or choosing healthy options:
*Leave the dressing off or use avocado/ cottage cheese/etc.
*Leave off bacon and fried foods.

*Put on extra vegetables instead of extra meat and cheese
*Share entrees with someone else
*Order salad or vegetables instead of fries and rings
*Have your entrée split in half and boxed before it arrives at the table.
*Order meat to be grilled or baked and breads to be whole grain.
*Choose an appetite portion or child's portion

Day 10

Restaurant Choices	
Restaurant name:	Menu choice with modifications
Restaurant name:	Menu choice with modifications
Restaurant name:	Menu choice with modifications
Restaurant name:	Menu choice with modifications
Restaurant name:	Menu choice with modifications
Restaurant name:	Menu choice with modifications
Restaurant name:	Menu choice with modifications
Notes:	

Food that is processed passes through the body faster than food made from the earth's bounty. It is this abundance of food that can add untold calories without a person consciously thinking about what is happening. When food is processed it allows us to eat it so fast that it hits our stomach before our chewing and physical satisfaction of being full has time to hit. This can easily lead to 1000's of calories without realizing. Then it digests so much more rapidly than the unprocessed food, that we are quickly hungry again.

So while eliminating potato chips and crackers from out nutrition may be a great way to help us to our goals, there is also a need for a backup plan for those who are on the go. When you are traveling it might be easy to throw an apple in your bag for a carbohydrate, but what about your protein? It's pretty hard to carry around a chunk of meat on a hot day. That's where protein drinks or bars can come in handy.

Meal replacements can be easy to carry and already fit into your portion size. They can give you accurate protein and calorie counts. They can be inexpensive. Be aware, because they are processed, they can also keep you from learning how to make healthy food choices. While the usage of drinks and bars should be kept fairly minimal, it is far more important that you get nourishment on time and within your calorie limits so that you don't feel hungry enough to overeat. Just read your labels to make sure your choice is healthy.

Often an 80 calorie item may be in a package with 2 or more servings. This means an 80 calorie snack may easily be double or more what you thought. If a packaged product, such as a protein bar, has 20 grams of sugar, that means you get the benefit of the protein, with the addition of 20 grams of sugar. Sounds like a candy bar to me. That's not the healthy natural sugar you get from an apple.

So if you want a healthier snack, you might choose a protein bar, with minimal sugar. Then finish by also eating an apple.

When trying new protein brands, either chill the drinks or heat them. It makes the taste of the protein more palatable until your taste buds adjust.

Fill out the NUTRITION FACTS in your workbook for several different foods you eat regularly. Note what a serving size is and what the nutritional content is vs. the calories.

Day 11:
Item:

Nutrition Facts

Serv.Size:____
Servings per container:____

AMOUNT PER SERVING

Calories ____

% DAILY VALUE

TOTAL FAT: ____ %
____ Saturated fat: ____ %
____ Trans fat: ____ %
CHOLESTEROL: ____ %
SODIUM: ____ %
TOTAL CARBOHYDRATE: ____ %
____ Dietary fiber: ____ %
____ Sugar: ____ %
____ Sugar Alcohal ____ %
PROTEIN: ____ %
Percentage daily value based on
2000 calorie diet.

Item:

Nutrition Facts

Serv.Size:____
Servings per container:____

AMOUNT PER SERVING

Calories ____

% DAILY VALUE

TOTAL FAT: ____ %
____ Saturated fat: ____ %
____ Trans fat: ____ %
CHOLESTEROL: ____ %
SODIUM: ____ %
TOTAL CARBOHYDRATE: ____ %
____ Dietary fiber: ____ %
____ Sugar: ____ %
____ Sugar Alcohal ____ %
PROTEIN: ____ %
Percentage daily value based on
2000 calorie diet.

Item:

Nutrition Facts

Serv.Size:____
Servings per container:____

AMOUNT PER SERVING

Calories ____

% DAILY VALUE

TOTAL FAT: ____ %
____ Saturated fat: ____ %
____ Trans fat: ____ %
CHOLESTEROL: ____ %
SODIUM: ____ %
TOTAL CARBOHYDRATE: ____ %
____ Dietary fiber: ____ %
____ Sugar: ____ %
____ Sugar Alcohal ____ %
PROTEIN: ____ %
Percentage daily value based on
2000 calorie diet.

Item:

Nutrition Facts

Serv.Size:____
Servings per container:____

AMOUNT PER SERVING

Calories ____

% DAILY VALUE

TOTAL FAT: ____ %
____ Saturated fat: ____ %
____ Trans fat: ____ %
CHOLESTEROL: ____ %
SODIUM: ____ %
TOTAL CARBOHYDRATE: ____ %
____ Dietary fiber: ____ %
____ Sugar: ____ %
____ Sugar Alcohal ____ %
PROTEIN: ____ %
Percentage daily value based on
2000 calorie diet.

Day 11:

Item:

Nutrition Facts

Serv.Size:____
Servings per container:____

AMOUNT PER SERVING

Calories _____

% DAILY VALUE

TOTAL FAT: %
____Saturated fat: %
____Trans fat: %
CHOLESTEROL: %
SODIUM: %
TOTAL CARBOHYDRATE: %
____Dietary fiber: %
____Sugar: %
____Sugar Alcohal   %
PROTEIN: %
Percentage daily value based on
2000 calorie diet.

Item:

Nutrition Facts

Serv.Size:____
Servings per container:____

AMOUNT PER SERVING

Calories _____

% DAILY VALUE

TOTAL FAT: %
____Saturated fat: %
____Trans fat: %
CHOLESTEROL: %
SODIUM: %
TOTAL CARBOHYDRATE: %
____Dietary fiber: %
____Sugar: %
____Sugar Alcohal   %
PROTEIN: %
Percentage daily value based on
2000 calorie diet.

Item:

Nutrition Facts

Serv.Size:____
Servings per container:____

AMOUNT PER SERVING

Calories _____

% DAILY VALUE

TOTAL FAT: %
____Saturated fat: %
____Trans fat: %
CHOLESTEROL: %
SODIUM: %
TOTAL CARBOHYDRATE: %
____Dietary fiber: %
____Sugar: %
____Sugar Alcohal   %
PROTEIN: %
Percentage daily value based on
2000 calorie diet.

Item:

Nutrition Facts

Serv.Size:____
Servings per container:____

AMOUNT PER SERVING

Calories _____

% DAILY VALUE

TOTAL FAT: %
____Saturated fat: %
____Trans fat: %
CHOLESTEROL: %
SODIUM: %
TOTAL CARBOHYDRATE: %
____Dietary fiber: %
____Sugar: %
____Sugar Alcohal   %
PROTEIN: %
Percentage daily value based on
2000 calorie diet.

Day 12/ Date_____
Good Morning
Read your motivation.

However is a powerful tool you can use in every aspect of your thinking. We project our futures with the way we talk. So when you catch yourself saying some thing negative, follow it up with a 'however'.

My face is so round and fat, however I'm getting leaner everyday.

I can't stay on a diet, however that is the past and now I am educating myself to follow a nutrition plan that I can feel good about my entire life.

Fill out the form WHAT AM I SAYING through out the day. Be aware of what comes out of your mouth or what you think. When you catch yourself being negative, add the however phrase to reverse the negative. Change your thinking, change your destiny.

Keep filling out you Energy output form for the week as you see fluctuations.

Try to incorporate a portion of carbohydrate and a portion of protein into every snack and meal with additional veggies at least one or two of the meals. That's high quality carbs (fruit, veggies, low fat/sugar yougurt,etc) and high quality protein (meat, nuts, eggs, protein powder/bars/drinks) according to your plan.

Some people use the new "MY PLATE", instead of the food pyramid, because it is easier to visualize. Be aware that it is simplified. The grains should be high quality whole grains if possible and less processed pasta type grains.

Others try to make sure snacks cover at least two food groups to cover nutrient needs and meals cover at least three to four food groups. This isn't always possible when you are on the run and your choice is a protein bar or a yogurt/cottage cheese mix.

Again...this is your life and your plan. Whether you are eating three slightly larger meals and two or three snacks...or whether you are eating five to six small meals...you are designing a lifestyle to meet your own personal habits. Enjoy the process of learning who you are.

Keep charting. This is teaching you to THINK about what you are doing with your nutrition daily. When you think about your choices, you can make the choices that enable you to change..

Day 12   **WHAT AM I SAYING?**

When you catch your self saying or thinking something negative, write it down with a 'however' ending. Make the ending positive and say it out loud.

_____

_____

_____

_____

_____

_____

_____

_____

_____

_____

_____

_____

_____

MY PLATE

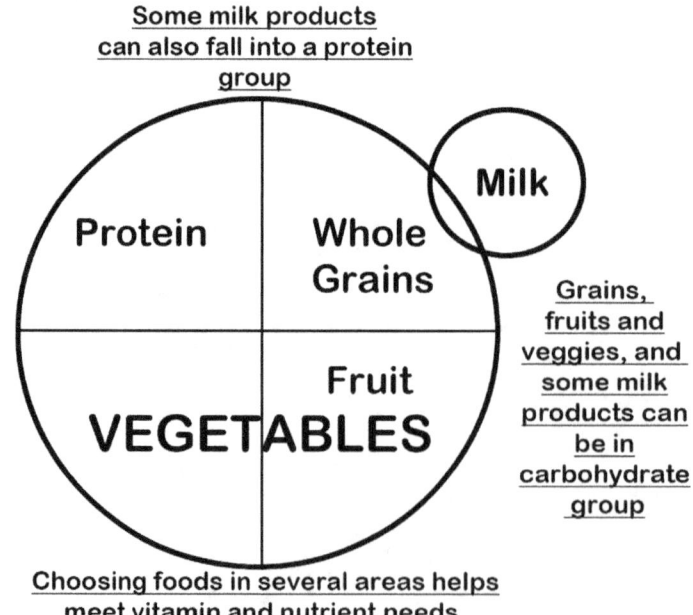

Some milk products can also fall into a protein group

Protein

Whole Grains

Milk

Fruit

VEGETABLES

Grains, fruits and veggies, and some milk products can be in carbohydrate group

Choosing foods in several areas helps meet vitamin and nutrient needs.

Day 13/ Date_____
Read your daily motivation.

Supplements and weight loss aids are some of the biggest sellers in America. So what do you really need?

If you are on a balanced nutrition plan, you may be getting most of what you need. However, many of us are already nutrient deficient because of the bad food choices we make. A person who is restricting their calories may need a multivitamin supplement because they have fewer calories to cover their needs. This is especially true if you tend to rely heavily on one or two food types and exclude other food groups.

When you work out, you add small muscle tears and injuries to your body that require vitamins and proteins to heal. Your healing is done at night, when your body is at rest. So if you are lacking a particular nutrient that will allow you to heal, you end up waking up without much good being done during the night.

A single multiple vitamin supplement can be a simple solution to making sure you have your daily requirements. This should be taken at night with a bit of protein so that your body has what it needs for repairs.

A simple way to examine whether you are getting all your food groups is to look back over your meals for the last week. Do you tend to pick up the same foods, or is there a wide variety of food that you eat. Remember proteins can be found in a variety of food groups just like carbohydrates can also exist in grains, fruits and veggies, and dairy. If you tend to eat a large portion of your food out of the same groups, you probably should consider a vitamin supplement.

Be aware that if you are eating processed 'fortified' foods with added vitamins, you may need to review what you may be getting already.

For the most part, keep things simple. Look for a multiple that covers the basics and isn't covered by a hard shellac shell, which makes it hard for your body to absorb.

As for other diet aides…you will find that as you become more aware of your nutrition, as you make good choices, as you stick to your plan…you will begin to feel better, have more energy, and start losing weight. There is no magic pill. Just the knowledge that the hard work you are putting in will pay off in health and quality of life. YOU ARE WORTH IT!

WEEKLY NUTRITION TALLY

Look back over the last week. Tally up
how many servings you are eating daily in
each food group This will help you be aware
of what you might be missing in your nutritional game plan.

Protein/ Carbohydrates

	Protein	Fruits/ Veggies	Dairy	Grains
Monday				
Tuesday				
Wednesday				
Thursday				
Friday				
Saturday				
Sunday				

If you find yourself lacking in a particular
food group, be more concious of balancing
your groups and think about taking a multiple
vitamin.

Day 14/ Date_____
Read your motivation.

While it is important to know if you are getting all your food groups and vitamins, it is also important to know if you are balancing your macro nutrients.

Fill out the **CHECKING YOUR MACRONUTRIENT BALANCE** sheet. You can plug last week's meals into an app program such as myfitnesspal.com. Then take your daily protein, carb, and fat totals and plug them into the worksheet. Multiply each column by the amount of calories that macro nutrient is worth.

This gives you the calories you are eating for each macronutrient. You can now pick which calorie range your day falls into, and see if your macronutrients are balancing out.

Don't let these exercises overwhelm you. The purpose is to learn a little bit more about ourselves and the food choices we pick. You don't need to do this as a lifestyle, but it's important to know where you are coming from to be aware of what needs to be changed. If you are eating so many nuts that your fat intake is top heavy, then you may need to save them for once a week or pre-package them into portion sizes before you overindulge. It's your life and you are in control. Make it count.

Day 14

CHECKING YOUR MACRONUTRIENT BALANCE

Protein-10-35% of daily calories
Carbs-45-65% of daily calories
Fats-20-35% of daily calories

MULTIPLY YOUR GRAMS BY CALORIES TO GET DAILY TOTALS

	Grams protein	x 4 calories	Grams carbs	x 4 calories	Grams fats	x 9 calories
Monday						
Tuesday						
Wednesday						
Thursday						
Friday						
Saturday						
Sunday						

1200 CALORIE DIET
Protein/ 120-420 calories
Carbs/ 540-780 calories
Fats/ 240-420 calories

1400 CALORIE DIET
Protein/ 140-490 calories
Carbs/ 630-910 calories
Fats/ 280-490 calories

1600 CALORIE DIET
Protein/ 160-560 calories
Carbs/ 720-1040 calories
Fats/ 320-560 calories

1800 CALORIE DIET
Protein/ 180-630 calories
Carbs/ 810-1170 calories
Fats/ 360-630 calories

2000 CALORIE DIET
Protein/ 200-700 calories
Carbs/ 900-1300 calories
Fats/ 400-700 calories

Day 15/ Date_____
Read your motivation.

Whether you have messed up or are doing fine, it is important to keep going. The more we learn about ourselves the more we will be aware of our actions.

Fill out the ACTIVITES OF DAILY LIVING FORM for 3 days. Give each activity the score assigned to that level of movement. Add your scores at the end of each day to estimate the number of calories you use on a daily basis.

This is a great way to see how active you really are and keep a perspective on what you eat. The accuracy of what you self chart and daily changes in habits can skew your needs some. While exercise can burn calories, it is often done in short duration when compared to daily activities of living. Building good muscle and raising metabolism is important to raise the calorie burning effect of the motions you go through on a daily basis.

Score sheet for Activities of Daily Living

Activity		Score	
	Sleeping	.8	
	Supine or reclining: Lying down, totally relaxed. Not sleeping.	1	
	Very light.Sitting and seated activities. Standing.	1.2	
	Light. Most light standing activities. dressing, cooking, bathing, clerk, regular walking.	1.3	
	Moderate. Brisk walking, jogging, cleaning, light to moderate exercise, gardening.	1.4-1.6	
	Moderately heavy; Moderate to vigorous exercise. Heavy manual labor such as digging or climbing	1.7-1.8	
	Heavy.Fitness activity such as cycling, stairstepping, or similar vigorous activity.	1.9-2	
	Sports. Vigorous sports competition. Football, soccer, etc.	2.1-2.2	
	All-out-training. Extremely high intensity weight training with little rest.	2.3-2.4	
	Extended maximum effort. Extremely high intensity or high duration sports. Marathon, triathlon, etc.	2.5	

Plug these scores into your 'ACTIVITIES OF DAILY LIVING' sheet to calculate your calorie usage.

Day 15

ACTIVITIES OF DAILY LIVING

Time	Activity	Score	Sub-total (score x time)

Total 24 hour score =_____

Total/divided by 24 hours =_____

Daily calories used- 24 hour total x 1,387 kcal =_____

Day 15

ACTIVITIES OF DAILY LIVING

Time	Activity	Score	Sub-total (score x time)

Total 24 hour score =_____

Total/divided by 24 hours =_____

Daily calories used- 24 hour total x 1,387 kcal =_____

Day 15

ACTIVITIES OF DAILY LIVING

Time	Activity	Score	Sub-total (score x time)

Total 24 hour score =_____

Total/divided by 24 hours =_____

Daily calories used- 24 hour total x 1,387 kcal =_____

Day 16/ Date_____
Good morning,
Read your motivation for the day.

Unrealistic weight goals or desiring to lose an amount of weight too quickly can result in rebound gain due to not being able to maintain a program that is too restrictive.

The National Institute for Health recommends:
     For a BMI that is greater than or equal to 35......
           A calorie reduction of approximately
           500-1000 per day from the usual intake.
     For a BMI that is between 27-35.....
           A calorie reduction of approximately
           300-500 per day from the usual intake.

Look over your last weeks menus. You can google basic food calories, or put your food in an app such as myfitnesspal.com. Find out about how many calories you are eating daily as a baseline. You can compare what you are now eating with how many calories your body is using. You may have been adjusting your nutrition and your calories are lower than what you are burning. If you need a further reduction of calories, add that into your plan.

In your workbook you can see an estimate of the calories you've been consuming to be at the weight you are. You can also see about how many calories it will take to be at your goal weight. By now you should also have a baseline of about how many calories you are using in your daily lifestyle. You can now make a determination of about what calorie range you want to stay in to keep moving toward your goals.

CALORIES NEEDED
TO REACH YOUR GOAL

Current weight   **Low   High**

[ ] x 14 =Low
      x 17 = High

[|]

BASELINE CALORIE NEEDS

Put in the calories
you used in your
activities of daily
living...Lowest and Highest

Low   High

[|]

RECOMMEDED INTAKE TO LOSE WEiGHT:
BMI greater than 35.....reduce 500-1000 calories daily.
BMI between 27-35......reduce 300-500 calories daily.

**You want to be able to: Have a program you will stay on
Keep you muscle
Lose your fat
So if you cut your calories a SMALL amount it will take you a
long time to get to your goal.
If you cut your calories a MODERATE amount you will see
differences, but not super fast or super slow
If you cut your calories a LARGE amount, you will see quick
results but you may be emotional, hungry, and unabe
to sustain it.
The ideal choice ususally falls around 20% below your
maintenance level**

Low   High

**Current weight calories x ,20
(Do for high and low range)**

[|]

**Calorie range for
moderate weight loss**

Goal weight

Low   High

[ ] x 14 =Low
      x 17 = High

[|]

**Calories to maintain
goal weight**

Day 17
Good morning
Read your motivation

We are now living much longer than we have in past years. There are studies in place that compare lifestyles of people who live to be 100 years old or greater. The only thing they found in common was exercise.

Aerobic exercise sends blood and oxygen to all parts of your body. The nutrients help with healing. It raises your metabolism and strengthens your immune system. Everyone needs consistent exercise.

Exercise has been shown to help with or lower risk of:

Depression
Balance
Early death
Stroke
Cancer
Diabetes
Heart disease
Cognitive function
Cardio respiratory

High blood pressure
Muscle strength
Blood pressure
Weight gain and prevention

Schedule your exercise times and days in your logbook calendar and keep your appointments with yourself.
Like everything else, exercise has to become a habit that you do regularly.

Day 18
Good morning,
Read your motivation.

Our bodies evolve, become stronger and adapt when we push them. A positive push can make your rise to a new level in all aspects of your life.

Being out of shape and having health risks was a push to get you to begin a change in your lifestyle. Now it's time to re-evaluate your goals and tweak your plan in any areas that are not working for you.

It's also a time to look at what's coming up in the next months. Take the time to plan an event, commit to an event, or find an event that will give you a push to get healthier. If you are slipping or falling off the wagon, get back on. This is about learning new habits and everyone falls occasionally. A 5k, family reunion, or getting dance lessons, will push you to stay focused and work harder.

Commit to staying in the game. Falling short doesn't count; only getting back on board. Believe in yourself.

Day 18

RE-LIST YOUR GOALS:

1)_____

_____

2)_____

_____

3)_____

_____

4)_____

_____

5)_____

_____

PLAN AN EVENT: (What is it? What will you wear? Where are you going? Paste on tickets, pictures, etcetera to motivate you.)

PUT A COPY OF THIS ON YOUR FRIDGE TO SEE DAILY.

Day 19
Read your motivation.
Good morning,

Americans have been increasingly exposed to larger portion sizes. Studies have shown that when people were given increasingly larger servings of food each day, they eat a larger amount without realizing the difference. Then, when the next meal arrives, they eat their normal amount without adjusting the difference. The bigger the serving the more we eat. The bigger the drink, the more we drink.

Often foods are packaged or delivered in restaurants that equal two or more servings. Looking at food labels or measuring can be a way to see what an actual serving size of that food may look like.

Having half of your restaurant meal put into a 'to go' box can help avoid consuming more than you need when away from home.

Putting a serving of popcorn in a bowl, then putting the rest away in the kitchen, can help with unintentional munching during TV watching.

Putting single servings on plates, instead of setting serving bowls on the table, can reduce reaching for seconds until the serving bowls are empty. Then clean the kitchen and leave the area to do other things.

Day 19

PORTION CONTROL WORKSHEET

1). Look over last weeks meals. Circle any meals that may have been 'SUPERSIZED'. (Large soda's, prepackaged subs, sandwiches or salads, restaurant servings, etc). Note how many times during the week this happens and how quickly an unnoticed trend may stretch your stomach and add to unwanted calories.

2.) Make sure you plan your meals for the coming week. Use containers to pre-portion your servings to learn what it feels like to stay on scale. Use small snacks or meals between main meals to keep your energy up and help keep hunger down when approaching the main meal time.

MEASURE YOUR MEALS FOR THE NEXT 2 DAYS:
(Write down what you ate…and how much a serving size is…such as ½ cup, 1 slice, etc..)

Day1:_____

_____

_____

_____

_____

_____

_____

_____

_____

_____

_____

_____

_____

_____

_____

Day2:_____

_____

_____

_____

_____

_____

_____

_____

_____

_____

_____

_____

_____

NOTES:

DAY 20

Read your motivation

BALANCING YOUR NUTRIENTS

Add two additional food groups to main meals.

Make meal, one hour before working out, soft food (greek yogurt, banana and milk, protein drink or bar, etc)

Make meal, within one hour after working out, more substantial (Sandwich, meat and carbs, protein drink, protein bar, etc)

WAKE-UP-DRINK WATER

½ hour before meal-Water

MEAL: Protein and carb from 2 food groups

½ hour after meal-Water

½ hour before meal-Water

MEAL: Protein and carb from 2 food groups

½ hour after meal-Water

½ hour before meal-Water

MEAL: Protein and carb from 2 food groups

½ hour after meal-Water

½ hour before meal-Water

MEAL: Protein and carb from 2 food groups

½ hour after meal-Water

½ hour before meal-Water

MEAL: Protein and carb from 2 food groups

½ hour after meal-Water

½ hour before meal-Water

MEAL: Protein and carb from 2 food groups

½ hour after meal-Water

VITAMINS BEFORE BED AT LAST MEAL. No water 1 hour before bedtime.

Before workout:

_____

WORKOUT

_____

After workout

_____

_____

DAY 21
Read your motivation
PASSING ON YOUR EXAMPLE
Look at those around you. Who (children, grandchildren, siblings, etc) have witnessed bad eating and exercising patterns and may be mimicking them in their own lives?

_____

_____

_____

_____

_____

_____

What behavior patterns are you witnessing in those you have been an example for? (Gorging, hiding food, eating disorder, sugar addiction, fast food, excuses not to change or exercise, etc).

_____

_____

_____

_____

_____

_____

WRITE THE NAMES OF THOSE YOU HAVE IMPACTED ON SLIPS OF PAER AND PUT ON YOUR FRIDGE. This is a reminder how important good values and habits are. You can not lecture them, but you can be a shining example of how important it is to LIVE good habits. Someday they may ask YOU how to change for the better.

DAY 22
Read your motivation.
<u>BRAG PAGE</u>
Time to forget about what you did wrong and brag about what you've accomplished so far. Lost weight? Eating more vegetables? Sleeping better? Exercising? Logging? Learning about nutrition? Getting back in the game quicker? Drinking more water? List 5 improvements that you have been working on and can pat yourself on the back about.

1_____

2_____

3_____

4_____

5_____

Notes for your self: What are some things I have learned about myself?

Day 23
Read your motivation.

SLEEP PATTERNS

Think back over your sleep patterns.

Do you tend to get up several times during the night?
   ***Practice being fully hydrated for 3 hours prior to bedtime, then nothing the last hour before sleep so that you can eliminate before bedtime.**
 Do you worry?
   *****Keep a notebook by the bed and write down anything that you need to deal with the next day. Then your mind can relax and rest without being afraid of overlooking anything.**
Is it hard to go to sleep?
   *****Practice meditation and deep restful breathing.**
   *****Write down anything that is bothering you to remember to deal with tomorrow.**
   *****Make sure your room is dark and you go to bed at the same time each night.**
   *****If your mind is stimulated by TV or Internet, try making a soothing bath or other relaxing activity part of your routine for the last hour of the evening.**
   *****Make sure you get regular exercise earlier in the day so that you can de-stress and be tired.**

WRITE DOWN ANYOTHER SLEEP ISSUES AND RESEARCH HOW YOU CAN PROBLEM SOLVE:

_____

_____

_____

_____

_____

_____

DAY 24
Read your motivation.

<u>PASSING IT ON</u>

It is important to quit being the embarrassed, out of shape, dejected person we may have begun this journey as, and give back to those around us. Your attitude may be what gives them the strength to be better themselves.

Find 5 ways, today, that you can pass on a willing spirit and helpful attitude. What can you do for others?

1_____

2_____

3_____

4_____

5_____

Notes: Think of other ways you can be of value to your community.

Day 25/ /Date_____
Read your motivation.

ASKING THE RIGHT QUESTIONS

What can I do today that will give me more energy?
_____

_____

Where, in my schedule, can I fit in a good workout today?
_____

_____

What is a fun thing that I can do with my friends or family that will be healthy?
_____

_____

What can I do today that will make me feel as though I am reaching my full potential and living my life with passion?
_____

_____

What's a great way to get my water in today?
_____

_____

What combinations of food, in my meals and snacks, can I enjoy today that will not make me feel deprived, but help my nutrition and give me energy?
_____

_____

Day 26/ Date_____

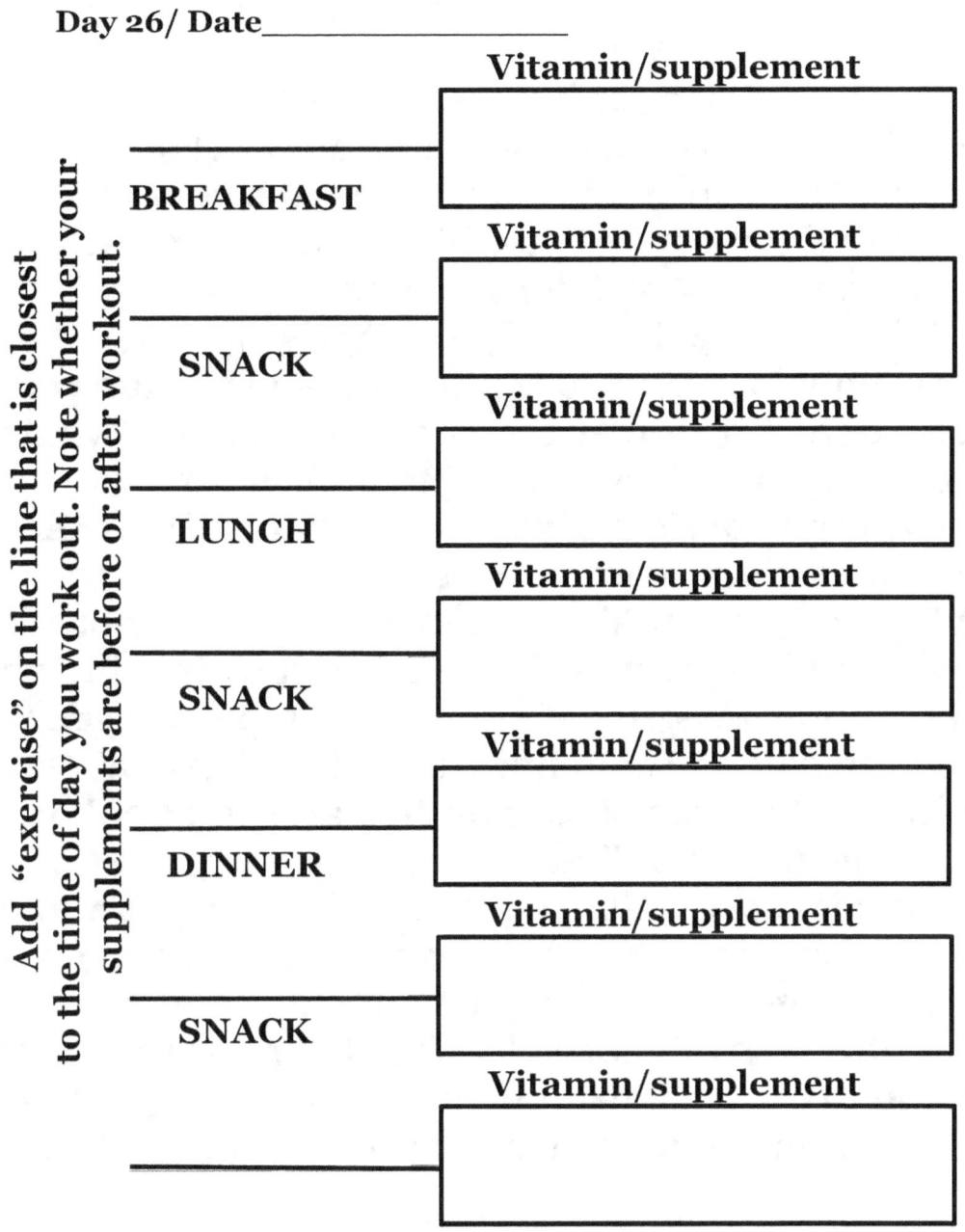

Vitamin/supplement

BREAKFAST

Vitamin/supplement

SNACK

Vitamin/supplement

LUNCH

Vitamin/supplement

SNACK

Vitamin/supplement

DINNER

Vitamin/supplement

SNACK

Vitamin/supplement

Add "exercise" on the line that is closest to the time of day you work out. Note whether your supplements are before or after workout.

Day 27/Date_____

Read your daily motivation/Write a list of things that make you feel guilty on a separate sheet of paper. (Anything from leaving a mess for someone else, to stealing something, or hurting our body). Think about how this damages your character and feelings about yourself. Then burn this list and release yourself from your guilt. Decide what you will do when the situation comes up again. And follow through.

BREAKING A PLATEAU

Your weight loss progress stops or slows when your calorie deficit becomes the same or less than what you are burning up. It is important to look at both your nutrition and your activities to determine if you need to add or take away from an area.

Ideally you began taking in 300-500 less calories when you started this journey. This makes it simple to cook lower calorie versions of things, or simply cut your deserts in half and eliminate the extra chips with your sandwich. Add in a bit of exercise and you don't feel the deprivation of a diet.

Now that you are hitting a plateau, it is necessary to adjust down another 300-500 calories. You can do this by adding time or intensity to your exercise and shaving your nutrition a bit more closely. Making sure you are pushing to build some lean muscle, with weight lifting, can cause your body to burn more calories just being alive.

Day 27

Clearing Our Conscience

Run off copies of this page.

Find a quite place…

Write down things you remember doing that makes you feel like a failure or makes you feel guilty.

_____

_____

_____

_____

Write down what you should have done instead.

_____

_____

_____

_____

Now you have a plan of action for next time. As you build character and practice solutions to put in place of negative actions, you will find you regard yourself in a better light and like yourself better.

Burn this page and the things you felt guilty about and look at this as starting again with a clean slate. You can put a weekly time on your calendar to do this and practice setting yourself up to have a better character.

Day 28/Date_____

Read your motivation

BARRIERS TO EXERCISE

The top reasons for lack of exercise (in descending order):

Lack of time (69%)

Lack of energy (59%)

Lack of motivation (52%)

Exercise is habit. And habits can take months to establish. When adhering to a program it is important to get back on track, as soon as possible, after a relapse. Deliberately putting some actions in place can help you to establish these habits.

1) Focus on the experience. Noting how good you feel when you exercise or how strong you are getting is a positive feedback when you think about allowing yourself to slip backward. Name three things you enjoy about the exercise process.

_____

_____

_____

_____

2) Ultimately it is your motivation to get you to the gym or outside to work out. However, those who interact with other members and establish friendships with others who have the same goals, have more accountability to show up and get their workouts done. The feeling of having a posse or

friend to interact with makes the workout seem less work and more enjoyment. Who do you know that you can currently work out with, or what type of plan can you put into place to interact with others? Example: 5k, use a trainer, invite a friend, make a habit of getting to know others, join a club, etc...

_____

_____

_____

_____

3) Make a decision regarding upgrading your goals and program. When you have a short term goal, such as biking somewhere for the day, or making a 5 mile hike, or getting pictures taken, you have a vested interest in being fit enough to get through it without feeling like you are killing yourself. What goal can you put in place to keep yourself commited?_____

_____

4) Reinforcing your commitment. Place small rewards and pushes along the path of your journey to keep your motivation high. Things like movies, pedicures, new clothes, and haircuts, are ways to pamper yourself and encourage you to reach for the next reward.

_____

_____

5) Looking at why you miss exercise sessions and your personal barriers..how can you plan your day to have the time, energy, or motivation to stay in the game?

_____

_____

_____

Day 29
Read your motivation

YOUR WEAKEST HABIT

While we all occasionally miss a workout or eat a bit too much, there are areas of our lives that become a habit of derailing us. We cannot rise above our weakest habit.

Figure out what your weakest habit is (overeating at a certain time, reaching for sweets, underestimating our calories, not planning our meals, not setting out our meals, not charting, stress eating, skipping workouts, etc.) Whatever this habit is…you will need special planning to overcome. Do you need to plan meals and do some special shopping? Do you need to get processed food out of your environment? You have to know and be prepared to give something up, in order to get to your goals.

WHAT IS YOUR WEAKEST HABIT?

_____

_____

_____

COME UP WITH A GAME PLAN?

_____

_____

_____

_____

_____

_____

Day 30
Read your motivation

You made it this far. Now it's time to reset your goals for another month and start again. In a three month period, your life will completely change. The season will change. You may change jobs. Someone may get married. Someone may die. You may take on more responsibility at work.

Life never stays the same. Even if you have the same goal, you may need a different approach to get there. It's not about how many times you fall, because we all do that. It's about how many times we get back in the game. Eventually it will become a way of life.

So re-do your goals for another month. Take the time to invest in yourself and keep going. You are worth it!